Low Carb Diet For Beginners

Delicious Low Carb Recipes To Lose Weight Fast Without Starving Yourself!

Volume 1

By Andrew Mills

Copyright © 2016 Andrew Mills. All rights reserved.

Legal Notice:

This book is copyright protected. This is only for personal use. You cannot amend, distribute, sell, use, quote or paraphrase any part of the content within this book without the consent of the author or copyright owner. Legal action will be pursued if this is breached.

Disclaimer Notice:

Please note the information contained within this document is for educational purposes only.

Every attempt has been made to provide accurate, up to date and reliable complete information no warranties of any kind are expressed or implied. Readers acknowledge that the author is not engaging in rendering legal, financial or professional advice.

By reading any document, the reader agrees that under no circumstances are we responsible for any

Copyright © 2016 Andrew Mills. All rights reserved.

losses, direct or indirect, which are incurred as a result of use of the information contained within this document, including – but not limited to errors, omissions, or inaccuracies

Copyright © 2016 Andrew Mills

All Rights Reserved.

More Books:

www.bit.ly/AndrewMills

Your Free Gift!

Thank you and congratulations on your purchase of this book and taking the first step towards transforming your life. I truly hope that the information in this book will help you and provide as much value to you as possible in beginning your journey to living a healthier, happier life.

As a token of my sincere thanks, I would like to offer you a **free gift.** Please enjoy a copy of my recent book, _The Negative Calorie Diet._ In this guide, you will learn exactly how you can EAT your way to losing MORE…

Check The Back Of This Book For More Details!

Copyright © 2016 Andrew Mills. All rights reserved.

Table of Contents

Chapter #1: An Introduction To Low Carb

Chapter #2: The Benefits Of A Low Carb Diet

Chapter #3: How Does A Low Carb Diet Work?

Chapter #4: Foods To Eat On A Low Carb Diet

Chapter #5: Avoid These Foods At All Costs!

Chapter #6: Simple, Fast, and Delicious Low Carb Recipes

Chapter #7: Your Low Carb Action Plan For Success

Chapter #8: Conclusion

Chapter #9: Review This Book

Copyright © 2016 Andrew Mills. All rights reserved.

Chapter #1: Introduction

Are you tired of trying different weight loss methods without any substantial or long-term success? Are you looking to begin the process of building a happier, healthier lifestyle for yourself that you can be proud of? Or, maybe you just want to be able to be able to feel great about yourself when you're around others. If it's one thing that matters the most in life, it's being able to enjoy quality moments with the people that matter most.

If these things sound like something you're interested in, then get ready to explore one of the most proven, trusted, and reliable methods of losing weight, and feeling great.

The low carb diet has been heavily endorsed as being one of the most effective solutions for improved health and weight loss for decades. Over the years, many diet fads have come and gone, yet the low carb diet remains a top option for many.

As the name suggests, the low carb diet is simply an alternative method of eating that requires you to cut back on consuming refined sugars and carbs. There are several different variations of the standard low carb diet, however the most common and effective among them is a low carb, high-fat diet (good fats of course!).

Once you get started on the diet, you should notice early success. Many people notice significant weight loss within the first two weeks of starting the low carb diet. This is the result of your body switching to fat burning mode once you are no longer relying on carbohydrates for energy. After this early success, most people experience a consistent loss of 1 or 2 pounds per week while sticking to a low-carb diet.

What To Expect From This Guide

To begin, you will firstly learn the many benefits of choosing a low carb diet. While this diet has gained considerable attention for its weight loss effects, it is also a great way to improving your overall health by reducing the risk of heart disease, diabetes, and filling your body with an abundance of energy. You will then learn exactly how the low carb diet works, and its effects on your body. Understanding how a diet works is absolutely critical to your success as you will have the knowledge needed to make proper decisions when it comes to food.

You will be introduced to a list of healthy foods that you will get to enjoy on this diet. After learning what foods you must focus on eating, you will be provided with a list of foods that you must avoid. These foods will primarily consist of refined sugars and carbs. Although, some of the other foods you must also avoid may surprise you!

For your convenience, you will be provided with delicious, easy-to-make recipes that you will be able make for yourself and your family. You will be so impressed by the taste and convenience of these meals, that you will become aware of just how simple it can be to eat healthy.

Finally, to ensure your long-term success with this diet, you will be provided with an easy, step-by-step action plan that will help keep you on track to achieving your health goals. You can be on any diet you wish, but if you do not have a plan or a guide, your weight loss efforts will not be sustainable long-term. This is why we will cover a couple simple things that you need to do to gain lasting results!

If you're ready to explore this new chapter in your life, then I encourage you to use this eBook as your personal guide to your own health and wellness success.

Within this guide, you will learn everything that you need to know to getting started on your low carb diet!

Chapter #2: The Benefits of a Low Carb Diet

The average Western diet consists of 3 large meals per day, with many of the meals based on complex carbohydrates and other unhealthy options. Over time, this can have a major impact on your health. You must understand that the reason many people are struggling with weight today is due to consuming an excessive amount of sugars and carbs. Any diet that is high in carbs and saturated fats can lead to an increased risk of obesity, heart disease, and diabetes.

By making some simple changes to your eating habits, you can increase your metabolism, start burning fat, increase lean muscle mass, reduce your risk of heart disease, and improve your health – to name just a few of the benefits of the low carb diet.

If you are on the fence about starting this diet or want to find out what you can get from this diet, then take a look at the advantages of low-carb eating.

A Very Simple Diet

Most people find that low carb dieting is not only very effective, but extremely easy to follow. Unlike other diets, your meal plans are not heavily regimented. This is not a complicated diet to understand or implement on a daily basis. The #1 thing you need to focus on is to increase your consumption of protein while cutting back on carbs. This will help promote lean muscle mass, which will strengthen your metabolism.

In order to follow the low carb diet, you'll just need to stick to a good selection of meals. Luckily, you will find a handful of tasty low carb recipes later in this guide.

You Do Not Need to Starve Yourself

Another great reason to consider following the low carb diet is that you do not need to starve yourself. Many people are surprised by the amount of food that they get to eat on a low carb diet. On this diet, you will be eating a lot of protein, which is very filling and satisfying. This will include three meals per day, along with one or two small snacks in-between.

Regardless of your previous eating habits, it is highly unlikely that you will ever feel hungry or unsatisfied while on this diet since you aren't eating less.

Low Carb Dieting Can Improve Your Health

As mentioned, the low carb diet can improve your health. It strengthens your metabolism and increases your cardiovascular health – offering a wide range of health benefits. Some of the benefits you will receive from this diet include:

- Strengthening your metabolism
- Promote muscle gain
- Reduce fatigue and increase energy levels
- Lower your risk of heart disease
- Lower your risk of diabetes
- Lose weight and keep it off

Strengthen Your Metabolism

At the core of the low carb diet is the ability to help strengthen your metabolism. You must understand that your metabolic rate determines the number of calories that you burn while at rest. So, by increasing your metabolism, you increase your natural ability to lose weight.

How does the low carb diet help strengthen your metabolism? Protein is a more suitable source of energy than refined or complex carbohydrates. By decreasing your intake of carbohydrates, your body begins burning fat in order to supply your body with energy. Today, most carbohydrate foods are extremely processed. This makes it very easy for your body to digest the carbs, which ultimately results in a buildup of excess energy that your body doesn't need.

However, since protein and high-fiber foods are more difficult for your body to process and convert to energy, your body begins metabolizing energy from your stored fat. Though, this is not the only way that the low carb diet can help boost your metabolism.

Protein is a necessary nutrient for maintaining and increasing muscle mass. With a low carb diet, your body will promote lean muscle growth. Muscle uses more energy than fat, providing a natural increase in your metabolism. Also, because you will be eating plenty, you will not be slowing down your metabolism. Eating plenty and not starving yourself is a key part of maintaining a healthy metabolism, which will lead to weight loss.

Reduce Fatigue and Increase Energy Levels

As mentioned, protein is a better source of energy than complex carbohydrates. After several weeks on the diet, you will notice that your energy levels will begin to stabilize to a healthy level. When your diet consists primarily of carbohydrates, your blood sugar levels fluctuate regularly. By cutting back on the carbs, you are supplying your body with a steady, more predictable source of energy. Along with stabilizing your energy levels, this will result in the added benefit of reducing fatigue.

Lower Your Risk of Heart Disease

Getting rid of unhealthy fats and sugar is great for your heart. Some people are weary about starting the low carb diet because they have heard that it can lead to increased cholesterol levels. The truth is, any diet can lead to increased cholesterol levels if you do not pay attention to the selection and diversification of food you eat.

With the low carb diet, you will be eating a variety of healthy sources of protein. This includes lean meat such as poultry and fish, instead of eating red meat which contains many unhealthy fats. By basing your meals around healthy foods and ingredients, you can limit your intake of cholesterol while still getting a great selection of beneficial fats for your body.

Lower Your Risk of Diabetes

As mentioned, when your diet is based largely around eating carbohydrates, you will experience fluctuations in your blood sugar levels. A spike in blood sugar levels will increase your risk of developing diabetes. However, a diet based on protein, fiber, healthy fats, and a minimal amount of carbs will help you maintain your blood sugar levels and ultimately decrease your risk of diabetes.

Lose Weight and Keep It Off

By cutting back on refined sugars and carbohydrates, you will also be cutting back on processed foods and junk food. You will be basing your meals around healthy, whole ingredients. This alone will help you lose weight, but when combined with the other benefits already discussed, you will likely have no problem reaching your ideal weight.

For decades, people have used low carb dieting to promote weight loss and increase their metabolism. This is a sustainable diet that you can continue to follow for the rest of your life! You can enjoy a healthy life simply by changing the way that you eat. Now that you know why you should follow the low carb diet, it is time to learn how the diet works.

Chapter #3: How Does a Low Carb Diet Work?

The low carb diet receives a lot of attention. You have probably read an article here or there about the diet, but do not fully understand what it entails. Most people understand that you need to cut back on bread and pasta, but before you can get started on a low carb diet, you need to understand more about the structure of how the diet exactly works.

Basing Your Meals Around Protein

There is a lot more to the low carb diet than simply cutting back on your intake of carbohydrates. You also need to ensure that you are receiving enough protein to compensate for the loss of energy from carbs. Otherwise, you will be depriving yourself of nutrition, which is not a sustainable method of achieving weight loss.

The majority of your meals will be based around protein. This includes lean meats, eggs, some dairy products, and any other food that are low in carbs and high in protein or fiber. You will work with a base nutritional recommendation for your daily intake of protein and carbs.

How Much Carbs Can You Eat?

For the carbohydrates, you should try to limit yourself to 20 grams per day. This is necessary for encouraging your body to burn fat for energy. As discussed, your body is currently used to converting carbs into sugar for energy and then storing the rest as fat. When you no longer supply your body with carbs, it will have no choice but to burn fat.

Once you reach your ideal weight, you will begin increasing your daily intake of carbs, eventually reaching around 60 carbohydrates per day. This will be explained in detail later on. For now, remember that you must try your best to consume only 20 grams of carbs per day.

How Much Protein Should You Eat?

There are several schools of thought on how to determine the amount of protein that you should consume each day. However, the simplest method of doing so is to multiply your weight in pounds by 0.37. So, if you weigh 200 pounds, you should consume roughly 74 grams of protein per day. Some nutritionists might recommend that you take into account your daily activity level, but this is not very necessary unless you lead a very active lifestyle and need to include additional protein to maintain your current muscle mass.

Later on in the foods section of this guide, you will find a list of protein-rich foods that you can eat to fulfill your high protein demands. These lists are not all-inclusive, but they will offer enough recommendations to get you started and to give you a general idea of the types of foods that you will be eating and the types of foods to avoid.

Chapter #4: Foods to Eat on a Low Carb Diet

What can you eat while following a low carb diet? This is the main question that many people want to know before starting any diet (and it's a good question to have!). One of the great features of the low carb diet is that you have a wide range of foods to choose from eating.

The low carb diet is not an overly restrictive diet, which can make it easier for you to stick to your dieting plans. Here is a list of different types of foods that you can enjoy on the low carb diet:

- Cheese – Aim to use full-fat cheeses, as low-fat options remove good fats.
- Cream – Full-fat cream contains healthy fats as well.
- Eggs – Any kind will do. If possible, shop for free range eggs.
- Fats – Olive oil and butter are fantastic sources of healthy fats.
- Fish – One of the best sources of protein, especially tuna and salmon.

- Fruit – Choose nutrient-dense fruits, such as various berries, lemons, oranges, and grapefruit.
- Meat – Chicken, pork, and lamb are all great options. Though, be very careful with the amount of red meat you choose to eat!
- Nuts and Seeds – Nuts and seeds are a good source of fiber, but they should only be eaten in moderation.
- Vegetables – Any vegetables that grow above ground, such as spinach, kale, broccoli, and lettuce.

The foods listed above covers most of the types of foods that you will be eating while on the low carb diet. Along with the foods that you should eat, you will need to learn about the foods that you avoid at all costs.

Chapter #5: Foods to Avoid on a Low Carb Diet

In the previous chapter, you discovered a list of some of the most popular foods that you are encouraged to consume on your low carb diet. Hopefully, that list helped you get excited about this diet. Next, you are going to find out which foods you should avoid while on the low carb diet in order to be successful.

The following foods should be avoided while you are on a low carb diet:

- Bread – There are low carb bread options to use as an alternative such as Melba toast. However, pay close attention that you do not exceed your daily carb limit!
- Cakes and baked goods
- Cereal
- Grains – Including barley, wheat, oats, and sorghum.
- Pasta
- Potatoes
- Processed foods
- Rice
- Starchy vegetables

- Sugar drinks – Opt to drink water, milk, coffee, or tea.

Essentially, anything that contains a lot of carbohydrates will need to be avoided in order to succeed in this diet. If you are unsure whether or not a food should be included in your diet, simply look at the number of carbohydrates in a serving. Since you will only be consuming 20 grams of carbohydrates per day, it should be pretty easy for you to know what you can, and can't eat.

Technically, during your day you can fill those 20 grams of carbs with any carb based food that you want. But, keep in mind that you should be making the most out of the carbs that you are consuming. By practicing good habits, you will be less likely to break your diet plan. Look for healthy sources of carbs, such as the foods listed above in the previous chapter.

Chapter #6: Simple and Delicious Low-Carb Recipes

Now that you have a better understanding of how a low carb diet works, you will need some recipes to prepare. The recipes provided below are simple, quick, and absolutely delicious to eat!

The following recipes will cover your breakfast, lunch, and dinner. Having a variety of meals to choose from will help you stick to your low carb diet and experience diversity in your meals. You can use these recipes to get started on the diet, but it is highly recommend that you pursue additional low carb recipes in the future to add to your list of recipes.

Low-Carb Breakfast Recipes

First, discover some healthy examples of low-carb breakfasts. The following meals are quick and easy to prepare:

- Broccoli and Cheese Mini Omelets
- Spiced Scrambled Eggs
- Sausage and Egg Breakfast Bites

- Breakfast Skillet

Broccoli and Cheese Mini Omelets

These mini omelets provide 18 grams of protein and 5 grams of carbs per serving of two omelets. You can prepare these in the evening and then have them for breakfast for the next several days as leftovers if you would like.

Ingredients

- 4 large eggs
- 1 cup egg whites
- 4 cups of broccoli florets
- ¼ cup shredded cheddar cheese
- ¼ cup grated cheese of your choice
- 1 teaspoon of olive oil
- A dash of salt and pepper
- Cooking spray or a small amount of butter

Directions

Start by preheating your oven to 350 degrees Fahrenheit. While the oven is preheating, steam the broccoli florets in a small amount of water for about 6 to 7 minutes. Once removed and strained, they should crumble into smaller pieces. Add them along with the olive oil, salt, and pepper into a mixing bowl. Mix thoroughly.

Spray a cupcake or muffin tin with cooking spray or line with butter. Spread the broccoli mixture along the bottoms of the muffin cups. In a medium bowl, beat the egg whites and eggs together. Add the grated cheese of your choice. Pour this over the broccoli mixture, until the cup is about ¾ full. Top the mini omelets with cheddar cheese and bake for about 20 minutes. The edges should be brown and the tops fluffy. You can serve immediately or store them for future meals.

Spiced Scrambled Eggs

If you're getting tired of eating plain eggs for breakfast, spice up the meal with the following recipe. This should only take about 10 minutes to prepare and 20 minutes to cook. Serves two people.

Ingredients

- 1 small onion (chopped)
- 1 red chili pepper (chopped)
- 4 eggs (beaten)
- 1 tablespoon of milk
- 1 handful of diced tomatoes
- Coriander leaves
- 1 tablespoon of butter

Directions

Start by softening the chopped onion and chili in a frying pan with the tablespoon of butter. Once the vegetables have softened, add the eggs and a tablespoon or splash of milk. Gently scramble the eggs as they cook. When the eggs are almost scrambled, add the diced tomatoes and a few coriander leaves. Serve while still hot.

Sausage and Egg Breakfast Bites

This is another recipe that you can prepare in advance and then serve for breakfast for several days. You can add your favorite dark green vegetables to this meal, adjusting it to your liking. This will make 4 large or 6 small square bites.

Ingredients

- 1 handful of dark greens (spinach, kale, beet greens, or Swiss chard)
- 2 cups of crumbled sausage (uncooked)
- 10 eggs
- A small handful of parsley

Directions

Preheat your oven to 375 degrees Fahrenheit. Slice the greens into thin strips. If you are using kale, you will need to remove the stems. Sauté a small amount of olive oil or butter over medium heat in a large skillet. Add the crumbled sausage. Once the sausage is mostly cooked, turn off the heat.

In a large mixing bowl, whisk the eggs, parsley, dark greens, and sausage together. Pour this mixture into a greased 8x8 pan. Bake for 20 to 25 minutes, or until the tops are crispy. Allow to cool for several minutes before cutting into squares.

Breakfast Skillet

The Breakfast Skillet is a quick meal to whip together in the morning if you're in a rush. This serving will serve four people. If you have leftovers, remember to store them in an airtight container and serve for lunch or breakfast the following day.

Ingredients

- 2 cups cauliflower (grated)
- 1 tablespoon butter
- 1 tablespoon extra-virgin olive oil
- 2 whole eggs
- 4 egg whites
- 1 cup shredded sharp cheddar cheese
- 3 green onions (chopped)
- 3 strips of bacon (cooked and crumbled)

Directions

Preheat your broiler with your oven rack positioned in the center slot. Heat the oil and butter in an oven-proof skillet over medium heat. Add the cauliflower and season with a dash of salt and pepper. Sauté until golden brown. This should take about 5 to 7 minutes.

In a large mixing bowl, add the eggs, egg whites, ½ cup of cheese, onions, and bacon. Mix thoroughly with a fork. Once the cauliflower is cooked, spread the cauliflower to form an even layer along the bottom of the skillet. Pour the egg mixture over the cauliflower. Use a spatula to smooth the mixture. Cook until the sides are set. This should take about 4 minutes. Add the remaining ½ cup of cheddar cheese. Place the skillet in your oven and broil until the cheese is bubbly – about 3 to 4 minutes. Allow to cool for 10 minutes before cutting and serving.

Low-Carb Lunch Recipes

It is easy to come up with meal ideas for breakfast and dinner. Most breakfast recipes are based around eggs while dinners are often based around meat. For lunch, sometimes you may have to get creative. Prepare any of the following low carb lunch recipes:

- Ground Beef with Sliced Bell Peppers

- BLT Chicken Salad
- Bacon and Egg Salad
- Chicken Lettuce Wraps

Ground Beef with Sliced Bell Peppers

Ground beef is not always the best option for your low carb diet, as it tends to have more fat than chicken, poultry, and fish. Though, you can still eat ground beef and red meat on occasion, such as with this tasty ground beef with sliced bell peppers recipe.

Ingredients

- 1 red bell pepper (sliced)
- 1 small onion
- 1 tablespoon coconut oil (or olive oil)
- 1 handful of spinach
- ½ pound of ground beef
- Salt and pepper (to taste)

Directions

First, cut the onion into small pieces. Place some coconut oil or olive oil in a frying pan. Fry the chopped onion for about two minutes. Add the ground beef and season with some salt and pepper. After cooking the meat for several minutes, add the spinach. Continue stirring until the meat is fully cooked. Serve with a sliced bell pepper. This serves one person, but you could easily double the recipe to make two servings.

BLT Chicken Salad

The BLT Chicken Salad is quick and easy and will serve one person. Again, you can easily double the recipe to prepare enough for two people. Another idea is to double the recipe for your own meal and save the second serving for the following day for your own convenience.

Ingredients

- 1 boneless chicken breast (grilled)
- 4 ounces of leaf lettuce (chopped)
- ½ a small tomato

- ½ a hard-boiled egg
- 2 pieces of bacon (cooked and crumbled)
- ½ ounce Swiss cheese
- 2 tablespoons ranch dressing
- Salt and pepper (to taste)

Directions

Start preparing your BLT chicken salad by grilling the chicken. This recipe will work better if you cut the chicken into thin strips before cooking. Arrange the lettuce on a plate. Top with the chicken and the rest of the ingredients. Season with salt and pepper and then serve. This makes one serving.

Bacon and Egg Salad

There is actually more to the bacon and egg salad than bacon and eggs. You will also add avocado and tomato to make a filling lunch. Just keep an eye on the amount of avocados and tomatoes that you include to avoid going over your carb limit for the day.

Ingredients

- 1 ripe avocado (chopped)
- 2 hard-boiled eggs (chopped into chunks)
- 1 tomato (chopped)
- 4 pieces of bacon (cooked and crumbled)
- Salt and pepper (to taste)

Directions

Combine all of the ingredients, but avoid stirring too much. You want to mix the ingredients, but you do not want to turn the egg and avocado into a mushy texture. Once mixed, serve in a shallow bowl or on a plate. This yields one serving. If you hard boil your eggs ahead of time and cook a package of bacon the night before, you just need to chop and combine the ingredients before packing this lunch for work.

Chicken Lettuce Wraps

Chicken lettuce wraps will require a bit of prep work. You may want to prepare these the night before and eat them as a cold lunch the next day. While there are quite a few ingredients in this recipe, it is still a simple meal to prepare. This should make about 2 to 3 servings, depending on how much filling you place in your wraps.

Ingredients

- 1 pound of chicken breasts
- 4 ounces of Shiitake mushrooms
- ½ an onion (diced)
- 3 cloves of garlic (minced)
- 2 green onions (finely chopped)
- 1 handful of cilantro (chopped)
- 1 lemon (juiced)
- ¼ cup of reduced sodium (wheat-free) soy sauce
- 1 teaspoon of chili garlic sauce
- 1 teaspoon sesame oil
- 1 avocado (sliced)
- Iceberg lettuce (for the wrap)

Directions

Heat a frying pan with some oil. Cut the chicken into small pieces and add them to the pan. While the chicken is cooking, combine the chili sauce, soy sauce, lemon juice, sesame oil, cilantro, and the green onions in a large serving bowl.

After the chicken is brown and fully cooked, add the chicken pieces to the mixture in the serving bowl. Place the mushrooms in the frying pan, along with the garlic and onion. Sauté for about 10 minutes or until golden. Add this mixture to the serving bowl and combine everything until coated.

Remove the stem from a head of lettuce. Peel the lettuce into cups and fill with the mixture from the serving bowl. You can store the leftover mixture in the fridge and simply scoop however much you want into lettuce when you are ready to eat.

Low-Carb Dinner Recipes

While breakfast is often thought of as the most important meal of the day, in many ways, dinner is equally crucial for sticking to a low carb diet. You can prepare a wide range of meat-based dishes, many of which will result in leftovers that you can use for lunch the following day. Most people do not have time to prepare a fresh lunch every day. Bringing a serving of leftovers that you can heat up at work will save you time and money while helping you stay on track with your diet goals.

Here are some great, easy to prepare low-carb dinner recipes:

- Cheesy Tuna Casserole
- Fried Chicken Breast Pieces
- Bun-less Cheeseburgers
- Easy Herb Crusted Salmon

Cheesy Tuna Casserole

This cheesy tuna casserole recipe will feed a family of four. This tasty meal will quickly become a favorite in your household. It is easy to prepare and is a great meal to save for leftover meals.

Just make sure that you do not freeze the leftovers. They should be stored in your fridge for up to 2 days.

Ingredients

- 2 cans of tuna (6-ounce cans)

- 4 ounces of cheddar cheese (shredded)
- 16-ounce bag of frozen French cut green beans
- 3 ounces of fresh mushrooms (chopped)
- 1 stalk of celery (chopped)
- 2 tablespoons onion (chopped)
- 2 tablespoons butter
- ½ cup chicken broth
- ¾-cup heavy cream
- Salt and pepper (to taste)

Directions

Cook the green beans in a medium pot and then drain. While the green beans are cooking, sauté the mushrooms, onion, and celery in the butter. Sauté until the vegetables are soft and starting to brown. Add the broth and bring to a boil. Allow the liquid to reduce by half. Stir frequently to prevent the mixture from boiling over. Season with salt and pepper.

Stir the tuna and mushroom soup mixture into the green beans. Add the cheese and then place the entire mixture in a 2-quart casserole dish. Bake for about 30 minutes, or until the mixture is hot and steamy. Allow to cool for a few minutes before serving.

Fried Chicken Breast Pieces

You need to be careful when preparing fried chicken. The following recipe will show you how to prepare fried chicken without adding too many carbs to the meal. This will make two low-carb servings of fried chicken breast pieces.

Ingredients

- 1-pound of chicken breast (cut into small pieces)
- 1 tablespoon of butter
- ½ tablespoon of curry powder
- 1 teaspoon of garlic powder
- 1 dash of salt and pepper
- 1 cup of dark greens (spinach, kale, or Swiss chard)

Directions

Cut the chicken breast into small pieces. Place the butter in a frying pan and turn the heat to medium. Add the chicken and then stir in the salt, pepper, garlic powder, and curry powder. Stir until the chicken is brown and crunchy – about 15 minutes. Serve with a cup of dark greens split between two plates.

Bun-less Cheeseburgers

Bun-less cheeseburgers are a staple of low-carb dieting. Just because you need to leave bread out of your diet does not mean that you have to give up cheeseburgers. The following recipe will teach you how to prepare a bun-less cheeseburger. Once you are comfortable with this recipe, you can then use this as a base to prepare your other favorite burger recipes. This will make one serving. Again, you can easily double, triple, or quadruple the recipe to prepare more burgers for your convenience.

Ingredients

- ½-pound of ground beef
- 4 slices of cheddar cheese
- 2 tablespoons of cream cheese
- 4 spinach leaves

- Salt and pepper (to taste)

Directions

First, form two patties from the ½-pound of ground beef. Season with salt and pepper. Place a small amount of butter in a frying pan. Cook the burgers over medium-high heat. When the burgers are almost ready, flip them once. Add two slices of cheddar cheese to each burger, along with one tablespoon of cream cheese. Turn the heat down and place a lid over the pan until the cheese has melted.

Place two leaves of spinach on a plate. Add one burger patty to each spinach leaf. Top with another slice of spinach of serve.

Easy Herb Crusted Salmon

Salmon is one of the healthiest meat choices. It is a great source of protein and also contains a healthy dose of omega-3 fatty acids. Use the following recipe to prepare delicious herb crusted salmon for two people.

Ingredients

- 2 salmon fillets
- 1 tablespoon coconut flour
- 2 tablespoons fresh parsley
- 1 tablespoon olive oil
- 1 tablespoon Dijon mustard
- Salt and pepper (to taste)

Directions

Preheat your oven to 450 degrees Fahrenheit. Place the salmon fillets on a baking sheet lined with foil or parchment paper. Rub Dijon mustard and olive oil into your salmon. In a small bowl, combine the coconut flour, parsley, and salt and pepper. Sprinkle this mixture over the salmon using a spoon. Use your hand to pat the mixture down. Cook for 10 to 15 minutes. You now have herb crusted salmon. If you prefer, you can serve with a small serving of dark greens.

You now have 4 breakfasts, 4 lunches, and 4 dinners that you can use as your base for starting the low-carb diet. Mix and match meals to keep things interesting and remember to keep your eye out for meals that are low in carbs and high in beneficial fats.

Chapter #7: Your Easy Low Carb Action Plan

The hardest part about any diet is getting started. While you could just jump right in and start preparing low carb meals, taking the time to plan and prepare for long-term success will increase your chances of reaching your goals. If you're motivated to make a change in your lifestyle, then make use of the following steps for your success:

1. Set a Start Date
2. Prepare Your Meal Plan
3. Include Moderate Exercise
4. Eat Leftover and Prepare Quick Meals
5. Do Not Count Calories
6. Set a Good Example for Your Family
7. Track Your Progress

#1 – Set a Start Date

Set a date to start your diet. I know this sounds so simple, but for many people the most difficult thing to do is to finally take the leap of faith and go for it. Plan in advance and mark a date on your calendar to fully begin your low carb diet without exceptions. You can start trying out some of the low carb recipes before your starting date, but once you start the diet, make sure you stick to 20 grams of carbohydrates per day, and other guidelines mentioned previously.

#2 – Prepare Your Meal Plan

You should plan out your meals for the first week or two before you start the diet. This will make things a lot easier for you in the beginning. If you are attempting to plan last minute meals, this is more than likely to lead to unhealthy eating choices which will tarnish your diet goals. Choose a selection of breakfasts, lunches, dinners, and snacks that you can use for the first couple of weeks, and stick to it.

Get rid of all your old food and stock your fridge with healthy options. By keeping unhealthy food in your house, you are only setting yourself up for failure. If you feel bad about wasting food, perhaps donate the food to a local food bank. However, by the end of the second week, your kitchen must be set for a low carb diet.

#3 – Include Moderate Exercise

It is always recommended that you include moderate exercise in your daily routine. Regular exercise promotes weight loss and better overall health. No, you do not need to exercise for hours each day, or kill yourself in the gym. However, it is highly encouraged that you start with some simple cardiovascular exercise in the beginning. Try to include 20 to 30 minutes of cardiovascular exercise at least 5 days a week. This could include something as simple as walking, jogging, running, swimming, or cycling.

While the low carb diet will help you naturally begin to lose weight, some moderate exercise can increase your chances of success and improve your health. Get creative with the ways that you choose to exercise. Remember, there are many sports or activities that are fun and great for your health.

#4 – Eat Leftovers and Prepare Quick Meals

You should never use time as an excuse to not eat healthy meals. If you have a busy schedule and feel that you do not have the time to prepare healthy meals every day, then make use of your leftovers or plan in advance. Plan meals where you can use leftovers from dinner for lunch the next day. For example, with most meat-based dishes, you can use the leftover meat for your next lunch.

You could also take care of some of your prep work for several days. If you are going to cook chicken strips for several meals, you could cut the chicken in advance and store it in your fridge. Several of the recipes provided in the previous chapter include cooked bacon and hard-boiled eggs. You can prepare these ingredients in advance. You could hard boil a dozen eggs or cook up a package of bacon. This way, you have bacon and eggs ready for tasty breakfasts and lunches.

Having a selection of different quick and easy recipes will help you stay on track as well. The recipes provided in the previous chapter are all easy meals to prepare. You can use these as a starting point for your diet. They will provide enough variety to help you get started on the diet. Though, you should continue looking for additional recipes.

#5 – Do Not Count Calories

The low carb diet is not a calorie-counting diet. Instead, you will only need to keep track of your carbs and protein. Counting calories can make it difficult to stick to your diet and requires too much planning and forethought. Not to mention, after all of the effort you go through to count those calories, you probably won't even feel full. Stick with the 20 grams of carbs per day and focus your thoughts on creating healthy meals that are based around high-protein and healthy fats.

#6 – Set a Good Example for Your Family

Starting a diet while your family continues to eat normally can make it very difficult to stay on track. Set a good example for your family. You do not need to force everyone to count their carbs, but by filling your kitchen with healthy foods that can be a part of your diet, you are encouraging the rest of your family to eat healthy as well. By providing healthy food options for your family, you are ensuring not only your long-term health but your family's health as well!

#7 – Track Your Progress

Keeping track of your progress can be a great motivator, but it's also the only way you're going to know if you are on the right track or not. When you tally the weight that you have lost for one, two, or three months, you can use your results as proof that you are headed in the right direction. It is recommended that you write down your weigh-ins in a notebook, on your calendar, or in your phone on a weekly basis.

Put these steps into action. If you want to lose weight and improve your health, you need to actually make changes to your lifestyle. Some of these changes will be easy while others will require willpower. Stick with it and refer back to these tips whenever you need a little reinforcement or reminders of how to stay on track.

Chapter #8: Conclusion

You now have the tools and resources that you need to follow a low carb diet. Remember to take your time when preparing for a diet. Before getting started on the low carb diet plan, you should decide which recipes you would like to try. Determine whether you are going to need additional recipes.

Additionally, there are a few other tips that could help you follow through with your plans and make the most out of the low carb diet.

Do Not Weigh Yourself Daily

You should avoid weighing yourself daily. Limit your weigh-ins to once per week. Before starting your diet, you probably already have an ideal weight in mind. Once you reach your ideal weight, you can wait one week and then begin adding more carbs to your diet. The goal is to create a balanced diet that you can continue to follow for life.

Start Eating More Carbs (After You Reach Your Ideal Weight)

After reaching your ideal weight, wait one week, continuing to eat 20 carbohydrates per day. Starting on the second week, add 5 grams of carbs to each meal – for an extra 15 grams per day. Every 2 weeks, add another 15 grams until you gain a pound or two. Once you detect a one or two-pound weight gain, reduce your carb limit by 15 grams.

You will then have a carb limit that you should be able to maintain for years to come, without gaining or losing unnecessary weight. The average adult should be able to consume about 60 grams of carbs per day without having to worry about weight gain.

Drink Plenty of Water

It is important to stay hydrated. This is true whether you are following a diet or not. Your body is mostly comprised of water. Proper hydration is the cornerstone of your health. Drink at least seven to eight glasses of water each day.

Do Not Give Up

For a final tip – never give up. One of the most common reasons that people fail at dieting is that they simply give up after a single slip up in their diet. If you find it impossible to resist a piece of chocolate cake at the end of the first week, do not use your slip up as an excuse to go back to your old eating habits.

You need to remind yourself of the reasons for starting this diet in the first place. Think about how great it's going to feel when you finally reach your fitness and wellness goals. Take drastic action right now, and make a change. Instead of waiting for several days or a week to "retry" the diet if you fail, return to your low carb ways immediately.

If you fall down, get right back up and try again. Stick with the diet and do not allow occasional food cravings to get in the way of living the happier, healthier lifestyle that you deserve to have.

Copyright © 2016 Andrew Mills. All rights reserved.

Review This Book

Congratulations! You have completed reading this book. If you enjoyed reading this, then I'd like to ask you for a small favor.

Would you be kind enough to leave a review for this book on Amazon?

A review would be **very much appreciated** as it will help other buyers on Amazon with purchasing this book.

To Review This Book, Please Visit...

www.bit.ly/LowCarb1

Copyright © 2016 Andrew Mills. All rights reserved.

Your FREE Book!

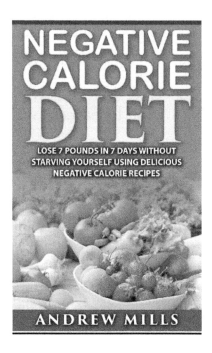

To Access Your Free Book, Visit…

www.bit.ly/NegativeCalorieBook

Copyright © 2016 Andrew Mills. All rights reserved.